Naturally Raising Your HGH Levels-

HGH Secretagogues, Exercise, Diet, and Lifestyle

Naturally Raising Your HGH Levels-

HGH Secretagogues, Exercise, Diet, and Lifestyle

....

Dicken Weatherby, N.D

Bear Mountain Publishing ● Jacksonville, OR

Naturally Raising Your HGH Levels- HGH Secretagogues, Exercise, Diet, and Lifestyle

© 2005 Weatherby & Associates, LLC

Bear Mountain Publishing
1-541-899-1522

ISBN: 0-9761367-0-8

This book is intended to provide information in regard to the subject matter covered. It is sold with the understanding that the publisher and the authors are not liable for the misconception or misuse of information provided. The purpose of this book is to educate. Information contained in this book should not be construed as a claim or representation that any treatment, process or interpretation mentioned constitutes a cure, palliative, or ameliorative.

Printed in the United States of America

Table of Contents

INTRODUCTION

Most of us do not appreciate the truly amazing blessings of youth until it is too late. The physiological signs of aging—weight gain, loss of memory and coordination, skin changes, sexual dysfunction, immune deficiency, low energy levels, and a general decrease in well-being—are often perceived as the inevitable effects of the biological clock's incessant ticking.

One of the reasons we experience these changes is the gradual loss of a substance called Human Growth Hormone (HGH). This is the hormone that is responsible for helping us burn calories, build muscular and trim bodies, enhance our immune system, boost our energy, and repair our tissue. It is directly responsible for the incredible growth seen in infants and children that takes a newborn to its full adult height and weight in roughly 15 years. Levels of HGH begin to decline as we get older and the negative effects of aging begin to creep up.

What if we could prevent that from happening? For some years now, injectible HGH has been available as a way to boost HGH levels. People get some impressive benefits, showing the power of HGH to halt and even reverse aging. But this method can have disturbing side effects. We will talk more about this later in the book. It is better to promote the natural release of your own hormones than to replace the deficit with hormone replacement therapy. Research in the field of hormone therapy has shown that the use of precursors, stimulatory agents, or secretagogues to increase the natural production of a hormone are often more effective and far safer than using the hormone itself.

And what if there were nutritional and botanical agents, and specific exercise, lifestyle, and dietary programs that could naturally boost the secretions of HGH in our bodies? Well, there are and this book will tell you all about some of the latest breakthroughs in the field of nutrition, botanical medicine, diet, exercise, and anti-aging.

Scientific studies have demonstrated that certain nutritional and botanical agents work via various biochemical pathways to stimulate the release of HGH. This is far safer than injecting synthetic HGH and allows the body's natural mechanisms to regulate how much HGH is being secreted. These nutrients, accompanied with regular exercise, and an "HGH friendly" diet and lifestyle, will increase the output of HGH and give you many of the benefits associated with a return to youthful levels of growth hormone.

This category of nutrients and botanical agents is known as secretagogues and in the following pages I will describe the basis behind secretagogues and what to look for when taking them.

It is not enough to simply ingest these exciting nutrients. They have to be delivered in a very specific way to optimize their use in your body. There are a few companies that are pioneering the latest research and development of targeted nutrient delivery using a very specific form of delivery called a liposome.

Before we get into the details of these powerful nutritional and botanical agents and the new techniques of targeted liposomal delivery, I would like to take an opportunity to discuss this incredible hormone and its effects on the physiology of your body.

CHAPTER ONE

WHAT IS HGH?

Human Growth Hormone (HGH) is a hormone produced by somatotropic cells, which are specialized cells of the anterior pituitary, a gland located deep in the brain. HGH is a protein composed of a string of 196 specific amino acids. It is the most abundant hormone released from the anterior pituitary with about 40 percent of the anterior pituitary gland being composed of somatotropic cells.

HGH, sometimes called the "Master Hormone" because of its role in the proper functioning of so many systems of the body, is really misnamed. It's role in human physiology extends far beyond the responsibility for growth from babyhood to adulthood. HGH causes the growth of nearly every cell and tissue of the body of the developing child and adolescent by affecting protein formation, cell differentiation, and cell growth. In an adult it is probably the most powerful anti-aging molecule in the body causing the cells of the body to regenerate, repair, and replicate themselves. I will talk about the profound effect HGH has on the body later in this book.

Unlike almost all of the hormones produced by the anterior pituitary, growth hormone does not interact with a specific organ, gland or tissue. Instead it has a wide reaching influence on almost all tissues and cells of the body. The different effects of growth hormone can be broken down into its physiological function and its influence on metabolism.

Physiological and metabolic functions of HGH

The physiological functions of growth hormone are involved with the normal growth and development of the body from infancy to adulthood. These functions begin to decline as we reach full height and size. The tremendous growth from birth to adulthood is due to growth hormone's impact on almost all of the tissues of the body. Growth hormone increases the size and the number of cells in the body and helps with cellular differentiation. For example it will help a cell differentiate into either a muscle cell or a bone cell. Growth hormone causes an increase in deposition of protein by the cells responsible for bone and cartilage growth, and facilitates the formation of specific cells called osteogenic cells that cause the actual deposition of new bone to occur. This signals the bones to lengthen until the genetically pre-determined length is established. This effect of growth hormone is most profound in the first 15 to 18 years of life. Although growth hormone no longer influences the lengthening of bone after the teenage years it continues to exert an influence on the repair of bone and cartilage in later years. Growth hormone continues to influence the deposition of new bone on old bone throughout our lives.

HGH's role in protein metabolism

Growth hormone enhances the movement of amino acids through the cellular membrane into the cell. Amino acids are the building blocks for all of the proteins in the body. Growth hormone also enhances the ability of the cell to synthesize and create proteins. It promotes growth and repair within the cell itself if adequate levels of energy, amino acids, and vitamins are present. Growth hormone causes a decrease in the breakdown of cellular protein for energy. In turn it mobilizes fat from the fatty tissue, which is used for energy, thus sparing protein as a source of energy. Growth hormone's influence on protein metabolism is almost instantaneous.

HGH's role in Fat utilization for energy

As mentioned above growth hormone causes the fatty tissue to release stored fatty acids, which are then preferentially metabolized or burned for energy. Under the influence of growth hormone the body "burns" fat in preference to proteins and carbohydrates.

HGH's role in glucose metabolism

Growth hormone has a number of effects on the cellular metabolism of glucose, the primary carbohydrate in the body that is used as a fuel. Growth hormone decreases the utilization of glucose for energy in the cell and increases the formation and deposition of a substance called glycogen

---

Summary of the
Metabolic Functions of HGH

The metabolic functions of growth hormone are not limited to the early years of growth and development but continue to exert the same level of influence into old age.

Growth hormone has a profound effect on tissue growth and fuel mobilization. It does this through its influence on all three of the major macromolecules of human metabolism: proteins, fats and carbohydrates (in the form of glucose).

1. HGH increases the rate of protein synthesis in all cells of the body.

2. HGH increases the mobilization of fat from fat cells in the body and increases the use of fat as a fuel for energy.

3. HGH decreases the rate of glucose use throughout the body.

---

in the cell. Glycogen is the storage form of glucose that is stored within the cell, especially the cells of muscle and the liver, and can be mobilized for quick energy. This may be due in part to the increased use of fatty acids for energy, which may cause the cell to shut down the process in which glucose is converted into energy. Growth hormone also has the ability to increase the secretion of insulin from the pancreas and causes a mild insulin resistance, which decreases the uptake of glucose by the cell. The mild insulin resistance is temporary and allows growth hormone to limit the muscle's use of glucose as a fuel and increase the use of fatty acids for fuel.

How does HGH exert its influence on the body? The role of IGF-1

Growth hormone is an anabolic hormone. Anabolism is the process of building within the body. It is the opposite of catabolism, which is the process of breakdown in the body. HGH exerts the majority of its anabolic influence through the formation of secondary substances called somatomedins by the liver. Somatomedins are the active forms of HGH that have a very potent influence on the tissues and cells of the body. Most, if not all, of the effects of growth hormone are a result of the formation of somatomedins rather than the direct influence of growth hormone itself.

The most important and most metabolically active somatomedin is called Somatomedin-C or Insulin-like Growth factor-1 (IGF-1) so named because of its mild insulin-like effects. Levels of IGF-1 in the body closely parallel the levels of growth hormone released from the pituitary.

Growth hormone is released in about 4-6 short pulsatile bursts across the day. Once growth hormone is released by the pituitary it is only around in the blood for a short period of time before it is rapidly taken up by the liver and tissues. IGF-1 on the other hand is released very slowly into the tissue and can be found in the blood 20 hours after its release. This greatly prolongs the metabolic effects of growth hormone secretion.

How is HGH production regulated in the body?

HGH, like every hormone in the body, is under the influence of an internal control system, which exerts its influence via what is called a "negative feedback loop". The negative feedback loop is not unlike the process whereby the thermostat in your house controls the indoor temperature. The furnace is triggered to turn on as the temperature in the room drops below the setting on the thermostat. The furnace continues to put out heat until the desired temperature is reached, at which point the thermostat is triggered again and switches the furnace off.

The secretion of HGH from the pituitary is ultimately under the control of specialized hormones produced by the hypothalamus, another gland located deep within the brain. The hypothalamus is like the master thermostat of the body as it is always sensing the changing shifts in hormones throughout the body. The hypothalamus produces two distinct hormones to help in the overall regulation of HGH levels in the body. One of these is called Growth Hormone Releasing Hormone or GHRH. This will stimulate the somatotropic cells of the anterior pituitary to synthesize and secrete HGH. The other is called Growth Hormone Inhibitory Hormone or GHIH or Somatostatin. Somatostatin causes the somatotropic cells to shut down

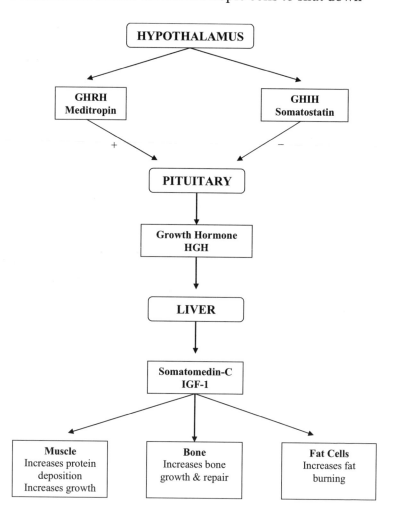

the synthesis of HGH, thus dropping the levels of HGH released into general circulation.

The hypothalamus constantly monitors the levels of IGF-1 in the body. As the levels reach physiological level it will release somatostatin and the synthesis of HGH decreases. As the levels of IGF-1 drop below the physiological norm, GHRH is released and the pituitary synthesizes and releases HGH. This is a somewhat simplified version as external functions such as sleep, stress, exercise, blood sugar levels, etc. also influence the synthesis and release of HGH.

What happens to HGH levels as we age?

As we age we begin to see a drop in the levels of HGH secreted by the anterior pituitary. This decline in HGH is known as somatopause. Levels of HGH peak in the adolescent years and gradually decline as we get older. Levels of HGH in our 60s are about 20% of what they were

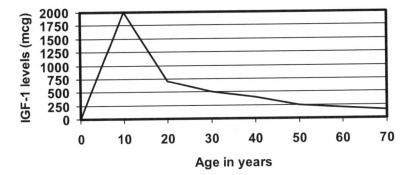

HGH Decline as we age

in our early 20s. The rate of HGH loss is roughly 14% per decade. The aging associated with HGH decrease was first noted clinically by observing patients who had an absolute decrease in HGH levels. Persons in their 50s who have been without HGH for a number of years will have all of the outward appearances of a person closer to 65 years of age. This is due to the loss of protein in the tissues, which is replaced with fat. The physiological effects of such a process are increased wrinkling of the skin, a decrease in organ function, a decrease in muscle strength, and an overall decrease in muscle mass.

Why do we experience a drop in HGH levels as we age?

We do not know the exact cause of somatopause. There is some speculation that it may be due to a number of factors including a drop in available amino acid precursors that are necessary for the actual production of HGH within the anterior pituitary gland, a decrease in the output of the stimulatory hormone GHRH from the hypothalamus, an increase in synthesis of the inhibitory hormone somatostatin from the hypothalamus, and a decrease in the number of GHRH receptors on the somatotropic cells in the anterior pituitary gland, which would prevent the pituitary gland from being adequately stimulated to produce and synthesize HGH. Each of these important factors are explained below:

1. A decrease in growth hormone precursor levels

As I mentioned earlier, HGH is formed from specific amino acids. A steady supply of these amino acids must be present in sufficient concentrations in the pituitary for the synthesis of HGH to take place. Amino acids come from dietary protein that must be adequately digested, absorbed, and assimilated to release their constituent amino acids into what has been called the "protein pool" of the body. Unfortunately our ability to adequately digest, absorb, and assimilate protein diminishes with age as our digestive processes in the stomach become compromised. Protein requires adequate levels of an acid called hydrochloric acid for digestion to take place in the stomach. The condition of low stomach acid, called hypochlorhydria, is very common as we get older. Hypochlorhydria is a side effect of a number of common degenerative diseases including diabetes, hypothyroidism, hepatitis, osteoporosis, and chronic autoimmune disease, and can be caused by the use of antacid drug therapy, the use of anti-inflammatory drugs such as aspirin, and is common in people who consume a diet high in refined carbohydrates, sugar, alcohol, caffeine, and refined foods.

Hypochlorhydria causes the available "protein pool" of amino acids to diminish as we age. It is not uncommon for an elderly person to have a 35% decrease in their available protein pool, which makes it harder for the body to synthesize specific hormones, including growth hormone.

2. Decreasing GHRH and increasing somatostatin levels

A second cause of decreasing HGH levels as we age is the decrease in output of the stimulatory hormone GHRH and an increase in the output of the inhibitory hormone somatostatin. This shift in the ratio of inhibition to stimulation moves in the favor of inhibition as we age. There are a number of reasons for this:

a. It has been shown that emotions, stress, and trauma can all affect the hypothalamus's ability to control growth hormone. These factors may cause an increase in the levels of somatostatin and decrease the pituitary's ability to be stimulated by GHRH. One of the main causes of this may be a decrease in the stimulation of a nutrient called choline. We will talk about choline at length later in the book, as one of the most potent stimulators of HGH production is a choline precursor called Alpha Glycerylphosphorylcholine.

b. High blood sugar may also be another cause for falling HGH levels. High levels of glucose in the blood significantly reduce GHRH activity and cause lower levels of HGH. High blood sugar levels have also been speculated to increase somatostatin levels, thus inhibiting HGH synthesis and release. Blood sugar dysregulation and type II diabetes are reaching epidemic proportions in this country

c. Another cause of falling HGH levels is stress. It is clear that people are under more and more stress nowadays, and this stress has a major impact on the adrenal glands. The adrenal glands produce a hormone called cortisol, which is one of the main glucocorticoid hormones. Normal levels of glucocorticoid hormone enhance the effects of growth hormone. However, excess glucocorticoid levels are released in response to the increasing stress levels. The excess glucocorticoid hormones have an inhibitory effect on HGH due to the stimulation of somatostatin release from the hypothalamus.

3. Decreased GHRH reserves

People also have a decreased reserve of hypothalamic GHRH as they age, which decreases pituitary stimulation to produce HGH. This has been shown to be especially true in obesity, as well as type II diabetes.

4. Decreased receptors on somatotropic cells

It has been speculated that as we age the somatotropic cells have a decreased number of receptors to GHRH on their cellular membrane. A decrease in GHRH levels coupled with a decrease in responsiveness to GHRH by the pituitary may explain another cause of the drop in HGH levels associated with aging. However, such changes are not seen with somatotropin, which continues to be synthesized and released in close to optimal levels by the hypothalamus.

Summary

It is clear from reading this chapter that HGH plays a profound role in human physiology and metabolism far beyond childhood and adolescence. The latest research shows that the drop in HGH as we age is multi-factorial. It is most likely a combination of nutritional deficits and environmental factors that change the receptivity of the somatotropic cells of the pituitary to GHRH and pushes the hypothalamus to produce more of the inhibitory hormone somatostatin than GHRH. This is like having a thermostat that is constantly setting itself to a low temperature causing the temperature of your house to be artificially cold. Increasing inhibitory influence placed on the pituitary will cause a decrease in the secretion of HGH. This will lead to many of the symptoms we associate with aging.

HGH Related Symptoms of Aging

Whatever the reason, the age-related drop in HGH is associated with a number of the symptoms of aging, which include the following:

1. Increased body fat

2. Decreased level of energy

3. Decreased stamina

4. Decreased muscle mass, bulk , and strength

5. Increased risk of osteoporosis: decreased bone mineral density

6. Increased risk of cardiovascular disease: decreased HDL ("good" cholesterol levels) and Increased LDL ("bad" cholesterol levels)

7. Decreased immune function

8. Wrinkling skin and graying hair

9. Decreased sexual function

10. Increased weight gain: reduced basal metabolic rate, increased hip to waist ratio

11. Increased depression and anxiety, and

CHAPTER TWO

WHAT ARE THE BEST WAYS TO NATURALLY RAISE HGH LEVELS?

Contrary to earlier thoughts, the somatotropic cells of an aging pituitary are quite capable of synthesizing adequate levels of growth hormone if given the correct precursors, adequate stimulation and prevention from inhibitory factors. Fortunately, the release of HGH from the pituitary gland can be restored using specific nutrients to stimulate the release of natural HGH from the pituitary. This can have a dramatic effect on reversing the symptoms of aging, leading to increased levels of energy, improved libido, increased stamina, improved lean body muscle to body fat ratios, tissue healing, and a decrease in wrinkles and graying hair.

Until recently these effects were only available to people using injectible growth hormone, which is extremely expensive and not without side effects. However, over the last decade we have seen a development in alternative methods of raising growth hormone levels naturally. These would include the following:

1. The use of nutrients to stimulate and increase the natural production of HGH from the anterior pituitary.

2. Appropriate diet to increase the output of HGH while decreasing the inhibition of HGH production.

3. Appropriate exercise to increase HGH output.

The use of nutrients to stimulate and increase production of HGH

The following section details the development of HGH stimulating nutrients from the use of injectible HGH to the latest developments from the bio-tech industry in a targeted liposomal delivery system.

Hormone Replacement Therapy vs. Stimulating Hormone Release

People who want to raise their own levels of HGH are faced with a number of choices. The first products available to raise HGH levels appeared in the form of injectible HGH. Oral HGH is ineffective because it is quickly broken down and rendered ineffective by the digestive system. Other methods of raising HGH levels emerged in the form of HGH secretagogues. We know that a number of factors need to be addressed before the pituitary can synthesize and release HGH. Firstly, the pituitary itself needs to be directly stimulated. Secondly, precursors of HGH need to make it directly into the pituitary gland, and thirdly, compounds and factors that inhibit the release of HGH should be eliminated (these include fluctuating blood sugar levels, adrenal stress and weakness, and stress in general). HGH secretagogues were developed to address these issues.

The first generation of HGH raising products - HGH Injections

The first method of raising HGH levels emerged in the mid 1980s in the form of HGH injections. The preparation of injectible HGH is obtained via recombinant DNA technology that uses the bacteria E. coli to synthesize Human Growth Hormone. This technology was initially developed as a treatment for dwarfism, which can be completely cured with regular injections of HGH.

In 1990 Dr. Daniel Rudman published a revolutionary paper in the *New England Journal of Medicine*. He showed that you could reverse the effects of aging by replacing HGH. His study selected a group of men between the ages of 61 and 81. Over the course of a few months they restored the levels of IGF-1 to those of a healthy young man by using HGH injections 3 times/week. The premise behind this was that increasing IGF-1 levels closely correspond to active HGH levels. Their findings were profound. These men reversed their aging by about 20 years. They also showed considerable changes in their body composition. These men did not change their lifestyle at all and yet there was an average of 8.8% increase in lean muscle mass. They lost an average of 14% body fat, experienced an increase in bone density, and reversed muscle and skin atrophy. Almost every system of the body responded positively to HGH replacement.

Given these remarkable findings recombinant HGH was soon widely used therapeutically as an anti-aging treatment. It is clear from the research that injectible HGH is very successful at reversing the effects of aging. However, it is classified as a drug and must therefore be prescribed by a physician. It is also incredibly expensive costing anywhere from $1500 to $2000 for a month's supply. The administration of recombinant HGH requires daily injections, which can be quite painful. The usual regulatory pathways mediated via the hypothalamus cannot work with recombinant HGH, which artificially replaces your body's own HGH. This can lead to problems with overdosing, reactions, and side effects.

The second generation of HGH raising HGH Products- Early Secretagogues

As the problems with HGH injections became known research turned to finding HGH secretagogues. Secretagogues are substances that stimulate the endocrine system to increase hormonal secretions. This prompted the development of the second generation of methods to raise HGH levels- the HGH secretagogues. Certain nutrients, specialized amino acids, and botanical agents were found that naturally stimulated and boosted the output of human growth hormone. When taken in a formula these specialized amino acids and botanical agents appeared to safely and effectively raise HGH levels. The use of such agents had the added benefit of allowing the body's natural regulation to take place.

Side effects of using injectible HGH

Over the years a number of side-effects have been associated with the use of HGH injections. These include the following:

1. Swelling of the arms and legs

2. Water retention and edema

3. Raising insulin levels that could lead to insulin resistance (an early stage of type II diabetes)

4. Development of antibodies against the recombinant HGH

5. High blood pressure

6. Carpal tunnel syndrome

7. Joint pain

NOTES:

CHAPTER THREE

NATURAL SUBSTANCES THAT NATURALLY RAISE HGH LEVELS

The latest generation of HGH secretagogues blends a number of specialized amino acid compounds and botanical agents into a broad spectrum supplement that brings a new way to enhance well-being and reverse the decline of health associated with aging. The next section lists the nutrients and botanical agents that, in my opinion, are the best way to increase your HGH levels.

An effective HGH secretogogue should contain a blend of the following:
1. Alpha glycerylphosphorylcholine (Alpha GPC)
2. GABA (Gamma Amino Butyric Acid)
3. Ornithine Alpha Ketoglutarate
4. BCAAs (L-Valine, L-isoleucine)
5. L-Arginine and L-lysine
6. L-glycine, L-glutamine, and L-tyrosine
7. Mucuna pruriens (L-Dopa bean extract)
8. Mumie, Moomiyo, or Shilajit

Alpha GPC

Alpha GPC is a specialized amino acid compound that has been shown to increase the secretion of HGH by changing the receptivity of the cellular membrane of the somatotropic cells of the anterior pituitary. It enhances the effects of not only HGH but every other hormone produced by the anterior pituitary, which include ACTH, the hormone that stimulates the adrenal glands, FSH and LH, hormones that stimulate sex hormone production, and TSH, the hormone that stimulates the thyroid.

Alpha GPC also enhances the synthesis of an important substance called phosphatidyl choline, which is an essential component of the cellular membrane of every cell in the body. Choline is also the building block of acetylcholine, which is one of the major neurotransmitters in the body. The synthesis of acetylcholine can be seriously affected as choline levels decline in the body. Choline levels decline as stress levels begin to rise and as we age.

One of the causes of decreasing HGH levels in the elderly is a decrease in the secretion of GHRH from the hypothalamus and a decrease in GHRH receptivity by the somatotropic cellular membranes. Alpha GPC boosts HGH secretion in the elderly by increasing GHRH output, decreasing somatostatin and by changing the cellular membranes of somatotropic cells thus increasing GHRH receptivity in the pituitary and increasing HGH secretion.

Overview of the Physiological Benefits of Alpha GPC:

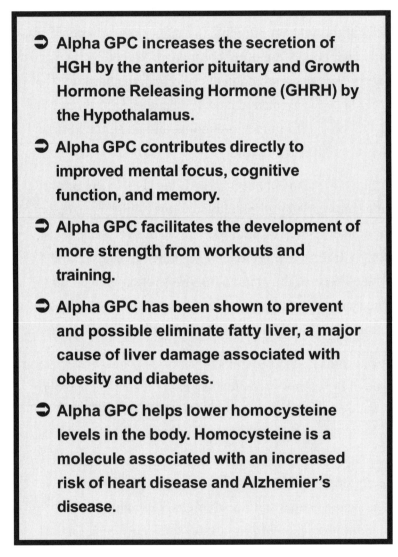

➲ Alpha GPC increases the secretion of HGH by the anterior pituitary and Growth Hormone Releasing Hormone (GHRH) by the Hypothalamus.

➲ Alpha GPC contributes directly to improved mental focus, cognitive function, and memory.

➲ Alpha GPC facilitates the development of more strength from workouts and training.

➲ Alpha GPC has been shown to prevent and possible eliminate fatty liver, a major cause of liver damage associated with obesity and diabetes.

➲ Alpha GPC helps lower homocysteine levels in the body. Homocysteine is a molecule associated with an increased risk of heart disease and Alzhemier's disease.

GABA

GABA is a specialized amino acid that acts as a neurotransmitter in the brain. GABA is broken down in the body into a metabolite called GHB or gamma-hydroxybutyrate, a molecule that has profound effects on sleep, especially the deep REM sleep cycle. GHB is a potent stimulator of HGH release from the anterior pituitary. Studies have shown that GHB causes an increase in the number of pulses of HGH released during sleep.

Overview of the Physiological Benefits of GABA

⮑ **GABA, via GHB is a potent stimulator of HGH release**

⮑ **GABA improves plasma hormone levels and has a regulatory effect.**

⮑ **GABA improves the body's sleep cycle.**

⮑ **GABA functions in the body to calm the nervous system.**

⮑ **GABA, via GHB stimulates protein synthesis and causes a release of fatty acids from fat cells**

Ornithine Alpha Ketoglutarate

OKG is a precursor of the amino acids glutamine and arginine, two amino acids that are strong HGH secretagogues. Use of OKG as a supplement has both an anti-catabolic effect (i.e. prevents protein breakdown) and an anabolic effect (i.e. enhances protein synthesis).

Overview of the Physiological Benefits of OKG

➲ OKG stimulates the secretion and enhances the effects of HGH.

➲ OKG increases lean body muscle gain and helps relieve muscle stress post-exercise.

➲ OKG has been shown to increase tissue repair by reducing healing time.

➲ OKG is a strong immune modulator increasing lymphocyte counts, improving the ability of white blood cells to destroy invading organisms, and stimulating the synthesis of immunoglobulins.

➲ OKG has been shown to increase uptake of oxygen by the brain.

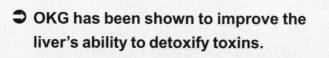

➲ OKG has been shown to improve the liver's ability to detoxify toxins.

➲ OKG has been used in cancer treatment to increase the cytotoxic activity against tumor cells.

➲ OKG improves integrity of the gastrointestinal lining and the overall function of the gastrointestinal system.

Branch Chain Amino Acids (BCAAs)- Valine and Isoleucine

Branch chain amino acids (BCAAs) include the amino acids leucine, isoleucine, and valine. They increase protein synthesis and have been shown to enhance HGH output. They are a useful energy source in an actively exercised muscle and have anabolic properties in exercising individuals. Valine is burned as a fuel and promotes the growth of new tissue. Valine and isoleucine work synergistically to promote lean muscle growth.

L-Arginine

L-Arginine is an amino acid that has a wide physiological effect in the body. Arginine is a well known HGH secretogogue that has the ability to stimulate the secretion of growth hormone. Arginine acts by inhibiting the release of somatostatin from the hypothalamus. Arginine also increases the response of the somatotropic cells of the pituitary to GHRH, thus increasing HGH secretion. Arginine has such a potent effect on HGH secretion that it is able to normalize the HGH response to GHRH in patients receiving chronic steroid treatment, which is known to inhibit HGH release. Arginine has the ability to totally restore the responsiveness of somatotropic cells to GHRH and inhibit the release of somatostatin from the hypothalamus. It has been shown that arginine alone is not as effective at raising growth hormone levels as a combination of lysine and arginine.

Overview of the Physiological Benefits of Arginine:

- ➲ Arginine stimulates the secretion of HGH by the anterior pituitary.

- ➲ Arginine is a potent immune modulator increasing the activity of macrophages.

- ➲ Arginine is a strong dilator of the blood vessels and greatly increases blood flow through the circulatory system.

- ➲ Arginine helps working muscles recover faster.

➲ Arginine increases the sperm count in men, improves libido, helps with erectile dysfunction, and increases sexual health in both men and women.

➲ Arginine also has a positive effect on tissue repair, decreases blood pressure, and helps decrease fasting blood sugar levels.

L-Lysine

L-Lysine is another amino acid and works side-by-side with arginine. By itself lysine is not a powerful stimulator of HGH. However, in combination with l-arginine it is very potent. A combination of l-arginine and l-lysine is able to boost the secretion of HGH as well as certain proteins from the thymus gland, which would explain the immune modulating effect of these amino acids as we age.

Arginine and lysine in combination have been shown to enhance bone growth. This may be due to arginine's ability to enhance HGH activity. Men with osteoporosis have shown an increase in bone density with treatment of growth hormone.

L-Glutamine

L-Glutamine is one of the most abundant amino acids in your body. It is another potent enhancer of HGH secretion. Thomas Welbourne, in his 1995 Study at Louisiana State University College of Medicine in Shreveport Louisiana demonstrated that a small amount of glutamine was able to raise HGH levels more than four times than that of a placebo. Glutamine can be readily converted into another amino acid called glutamate, a substance that stimulates the synthesis and release of GHRH from the hypothalamus, thus stimulating the pituitary to release growth hormone. Glutamine supplementation is a potent way to reverse one of the causes of diminishing HGH levels as we age. The neurons of the hypothalamus are very receptive to glutamine. By increasing the concentration of glutamine in the hypothalamus you will raise GHRH secretion.

Overview of the Physiological Benefits of Glutamine

> ➲ Glutamine increases the secretion of GHRH from the hypothalamus and stimulates the secretion of HGH.
>
> ➲ Glutamine increases mental alertness, clarity of thought, and mood.

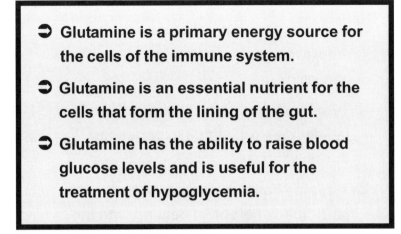

> ⮩ Glutamine is a primary energy source for the cells of the immune system.
>
> ⮩ Glutamine is an essential nutrient for the cells that form the lining of the gut.
>
> ⮩ Glutamine has the ability to raise blood glucose levels and is useful for the treatment of hypoglycemia.

L-Tyrosine:

L-Tyrosine is the amino acid used by the body as a precursor in the synthesis of three very important neurotransmitters: epinephrine, norepinephrine and dopamine, which are involved in maintaining mood, mental function, and sex drive. These neurotransmitters also have a beneficial effect of stimulating the release of HGH.

Overview of the Physiological Benefits of L-Tyrosine

> ⮩ Tyrosine is essential for the synthesis of the hormone thyroxine, which is the principle hormone synthesized and released from the thyroid gland.

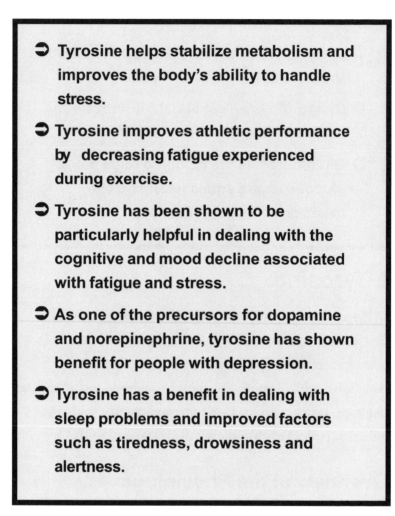

- ➲ Tyrosine helps stabilize metabolism and improves the body's ability to handle stress.
- ➲ Tyrosine improves athletic performance by decreasing fatigue experienced during exercise.
- ➲ Tyrosine has been shown to be particularly helpful in dealing with the cognitive and mood decline associated with fatigue and stress.
- ➲ As one of the precursors for dopamine and norepinephrine, tyrosine has shown benefit for people with depression.
- ➲ Tyrosine has a benefit in dealing with sleep problems and improved factors such as tiredness, drowsiness and alertness.

L-Glycine

L-Glycine is another amino acid that has been shown to be a potent stimulator of HGH production by directly stimulating the pituitary to secrete HGH. Glycine's ability to boost HGH levels is most readily seen post exercise.

Overview of the Physiological Benefits of L-Glycine

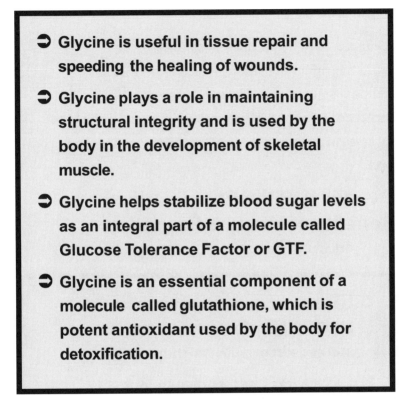

➲ Glycine is useful in tissue repair and speeding the healing of wounds.

➲ Glycine plays a role in maintaining structural integrity and is used by the body in the development of skeletal muscle.

➲ Glycine helps stabilize blood sugar levels as an integral part of a molecule called Glucose Tolerance Factor or GTF.

➲ Glycine is an essential component of a molecule called glutathione, which is potent antioxidant used by the body for detoxification.

Mucuna pruriens (l-dopa bean)

Mucuna pruriens is an herb with a long tradition of use in Ayurvedic medicine in India. Mucuna is the richest natural source of a substance called L-dopa. Mucuna pruriens has been shown to increase HGH because L-dopa induces the hypothalamus to release GHRH. We know that certain conditions in the body; including obesity, hypothyroidism,

Land diabetes can cause a drop in GHRH from the hypothalamus which leads to a decreased HGH secretion. L-dopa may be able to reverse that by increasing GHRH secretion.

L-dopa is used by the body to synthesize the neurotransmitter dopamine, which is an essential neurotransmitter in the brain. Dopamine facilitates the transfer of information between the neurons in the brain, helps regulate muscle control, immune function, and sex drive.

Overview of the Physiological Benefits of Mucuna Pruriens

➲ **Dopamine crosses into the anterior pituitary gland where it causes an increase in growth hormone output.**

➲ **L-dopa has been shown to increase libido and boost testosterone release in both men and women.**

➲ **Mucuna pruriens has an anti-diabetic function due to its ability to decrease serum blood glucose levels.**

➲ **Mucuna pruriens has strong antioxidant properties, especially for fats.**

Mumie, Moomiyo, or Shilajit

Mumie is a natural substance that consists of more than 50 different elements. Found in the Himalayas and the Ural mountains in Russia, mumie has been used as an anti-stress agent in Russia and India for generations. Mumie has a long history of use in Ayurvedic medicine for its ability to reverse aging and for its rejuvenating properties.

Overview of the Physiological Benefits of Mumie

➲ Mumie has been used for many years to increase strength. Mumie increases lean muscle mass, speeds up recovery of muscle tissue, and improves post-exercise recovery time in muscle, bone and nerves.

➲ Mumie has been used as a remedy for dealing with the declining mental function associated with aging. It has the ability to increase memory and has been used to treat dementia and other memory deficits.

➲ Mumie regulates protein metabolism, promoting muscle and bone growth.

➲ Mumie has been used for centuries to treat arthritis and as a natural anti-inflammatory.

➲ Mumie is effective for treating allergies. It has the ability to stabilize specific cells of the body that are involved in allergic reactions.

➲ Mumie enhances the immune system of the body and increases the cytotoxic or tumor-killing effects of lymphocytes.

➲ Mumie helps balance blood sugar levels by improving the secretion of insulin.

➲ Mumie has also been used as a remedy to improve recovery following both chronic and acute illness.

The Limitations of 2nd Generation Secretagogues

One can appreciate that these nutrients have a strong influence on HGH production and secretion, as well as a myriad of other beneficial properties. These ingredients are found in a number of HGH products that fall into this second generation category of HGH secretagogues. However, the effectiveness of taking these products in an oral form appears to be compromised by having to pass through the digestive tract and the liver before making their way to the pituitary. In my opinion many of the available HGH secretagogues fail to adequately stimulate or deliver key nutrients to the pituitary gland because they lack an effective delivery system. This has led to the development of what are known as the third generation of HGH secretagogues.

CHAPTER FOUR

ADVANCES IN HGH SCIENCE - TARGETED LIPOSOMAL DELIVERY

The lack of effectiveness of the oral forms of secretagogues led to the research and development of the third generation of HGH products, which are secretagogues that use a unique advanced liposomal complex coupled with a targeted delivery system. This method bypasses the digestive tract and the liver to deliver the key nutrients and stimulation directly to the pituitary where they are needed.

What is a liposome?

A liposome is a microscopic, fluid-filled vesicle whose walls are made of phospholipids, which are identical to the phospholipids that make up every cell in the body. Liposomes are used clinically to deliver drugs, vaccines, enzymes, and now nutrients into the body. Water soluble medications and nutrients can be placed in the middle of the liposome where they can be transported around the body until they find their target tissue. Liposomes have the natural ability to interact with cells and can fuse themselves to cellular membranes and release their contents directly into the cell.

What do we mean by targeted liposomal delivery?

It is well documented that biological cellular material can be attached to the outside of liposomes. The latest development in HGH secretagogues utilizes advancements in this field of bio-technology to put a unique biological "key" onto the outside of the liposome. The biological "key" that is used is specific for receptors on pituitary cells. The targeted liposome travels through the body in the blood stream and will only fuse with cells of the pituitary that have the correct "lock" for the targeted "key". This technology greatly increases the effectiveness of HGH secretagogues because the key nutrients that stimulate the pituitary and act as precursors for HGH synthesis are delivered directly to the target tissue and do not rely on the digestive system and the liver for digestion and assimilation. This technology is the latest advancement being used in cancer treatment.

Some research on third generation HGH products

This method of naturally raising HGH levels has been well documented. A study was done with 16 men and women to see if targeted liposomal delivery of HGH secretagogues would raise the levels of IGF-1 in a 30-day period. The results showed a significant increase in IGF-1:

- There was an average of 25% increase in IGF-1 levels after a month of using this type of targeted delivery.

- Changes in IGF-1 levels were greater for those participants that started with lower levels of IGF-1.

- The average change in IGF-1 levels was greater for women than men

- The IGF-1 levels were greater for those with lower body weight.

- There were no appreciable side-effects noted.

What are the main advantages of using these third generation products?

The direct liposomal stimulation targets the pituitary to release its stores of HGH and the key nutrients and precursors cause the pituitary to increase HGH synthesis. By combining specialized amino acids and botanical agents in a targeted liposomal form, the pituitary gland can be directly stimulated to synthesize and release more HGH.

Advantages of Liposomal Delivery
1. A liposome maintains ingredients in a concentrated form for increased nutrient density and stability.
2. A liposome is ideal for maximum delivery of ingredients to the targeted cell.

Benefits of Increasing HGH Levels

Increasing and restoring HGH levels to those of a teenager has shown to have the following benefits:

1. Increase lean body muscle

2. Decrease body fat

3. Raise energy levels and increase vitality

4. Enhance immune function

5. Improve sexual performance and libido

6. Increase cardiac output

7. Increase capacity for exercise

8. Improve skin elasticity

9. Remove wrinkles and eliminate cellulite

10. Improve vision

11. Increase memory retention

12. Improve quality of sleep

13. Lower blood pressure

14. Improve cholesterol profile (raise HDL and lower LDL)

15. Increase bone mass

CHAPTER FIVE

FREQUENTLY ASKED QUESTIONS ABOUT NATURALLY RAISING HGH LEVELS

What should I look for in selecting an HGH secretogogue?

1. Choose a product that has a reliable and well researched delivery method. My choice would be to look for a product that has a liposomal targeted delivery system.

2. Choose a product that has a mix of nutrients that both stimulate the pituitary to release HGH and also act as precursors for HGH production. As mentioned above, the problem with declining HGH levels is closely associated with the following:

   a. a decrease in the ability of the pituitary to be stimulated by GHRH.

   b. a decrease in HGH precursors.

   c. the presence of factors that have been shown to increase output of somatostatin: blood sugar dysregulation, high carbohydrate diets, lack of exercise, presence of increased levels of stress.

Choose a product that acts against factors a and b, and choose a lifestyle that acts against factor c. More on this in the next section.

3. Choose a reputable company that has a phone number where you can speak to someone who can educate you about what you are taking. There are hundreds of companies based solely on the web that sell products with grand sounding names, but have no customer support.

4. Has the product shown that it can raise HGH levels? Many of the companies out there rely on the original research that Dr. Rudman did on injectible HGH and apply that to their product. Call the company up and ask to see a copy of some research showing that it can raise HGH levels.

5. What are the fillers or preservatives? How is their particular product is packaged? This not such a problem for the oral preparations which usually come in capsule form or as a powder. However, this is more of a problem in the liposomal preparations, which have to be stabilized to protect the liposomal complex. Some of the liposomal complexes use substances such as sodium benzoate, potassium sorbate, and methylparaben as preservatives and to prevent degradation of the ingredients. It is important to remember that these substances are used to protect the liposome and are therefore not inside the liposomal complex, and the amounts used are extremely small. Both potassium sorbate and sodium benzoate are found in nature and are readily and safely metabolized by the body.

Research has shown that orally ingested methylparaben is rapidly metabolized by the digestive process, and is readily and safely cleared from the body by the liver. To put this into perspective, you would consume more sodium benzoate and methylparaben eating a few organic prunes or berries, or baking with cinnamon than from using a month's supply of HGH secretogogue.

What is the best way to take one of the newer targeted liposomal delivery products?

It is best to take any HGH product last thing at night and first thing in the morning. This mimics the natural output of HGH from the pituitary and gives you the best opportunity to positively influence your HGH levels. It is best to have a full dose at night and a half dose in the morning, unless you are over 200 pounds in which case you should take a full dose at night and in the morning.

It is best to take all of the HGH secretagogues away from food, drink, chewing gum, cigarettes, chewing tobacco, and toothpaste. The aim is to maximize absorption through the sublingual mucosa, and all of the above will interfere with absorption. It is best to take an oral formula on an empty stomach to increase absorption. They can also be taken one hour prior to exercise. As we mentioned above, exercise is a strong stimulator of HGH.

Do I need to cycle when taking these products?

Cycling, for those of you who do not know what that is, involves using an HGH product for 3 weeks and then taking a week off. No, you do not need to cycle with the HGH secretagogues. The idea of cycling an HGH product came about with the injectible HGH, and was designed to give the body a rest in between therapeutic doses of HGH. HGH secretagogues allow the body's natural regulatory mechanisms to operate, and therefore we do not need to impose an artificial regulation on our bodies by cycling.

Is there a cancer risk taking HGH secretagogues or naturally raising my HGH levels?

Human Growth Hormone is what is called an anabolic hormone that increases tissue growth and repair, and as such may influence the growth of cancer cells if they are present in the body. However, there is no inherent risk that increasing your HGH levels by stimulating the natural output of HGH from the pituitary will increase your risk for cancer because you are only increasing your own natural output and not supplementing with the actual hormone. Secretagogues, unlike injectible HGH, allow the natural control mechanisms to operate within the body.

Are there any other side effects of taking an HGH secretogogue?

HGH secretagogues are extremely safe because the natural regulation of HGH levels is allowed to function normally. However, a small number of people find the HGH secretogogue product to be quite stimulating and have to decrease their night-time dose to prevent being kept awake at night. I am not sure of the reason for this, but I think that it has a lot to do with the health of the adrenal glands, dysregulation in the natural cortisol rhythm, and the presence of blood sugar dysregulation.

If you find an HGH secretagogue to be quite stimulating at night you may want to look at your diet to make sure that you are eating the correct ratios of proteins and carbohydrates, and minimize your intake of refined sugars. Look at the amount of stress in your life, and make sure you are getting adequate rest.

Who should naturally raise their HGH levels?

It is generally believed that anyone over the age of 40 could benefit from naturally raising their HGH levels either with an HGH enhancing secretogogue product, exercise or diet. I think that it is best to begin the stimulation before your pituitary gets too affected by aging. This is different for different people, so use your judgment as to whether or not you are experiencing some of the signs and symptoms of low HGH levels and could benefit from naturally boosting your HGH levels.

There are individuals who would almost certainly benefit by taking an HGH secretogogue and following the exercise recommendations and HGH friendly diet because of certain conditions or surgeries they've had. This includes the following:

1. Women who have had full or partial hysterectomies during their reproductive years could definitely benefit from increasing HGH levels.

2. People who are obese or are overweight. The fat burning effects of HGH make this a must for people with weight problems.

3. People with chronic degenerative diseases (arthritis, auto-immune diseases, multiple sclerosis etc.) are often in a lot of pain and experience above average levels of inflammation in their body. It would be a tremendous benefit to naturally raise HGH levels in these individuals.

4. People who are post surgery or trauma would benefit from the increased tissue growth and repair provided by increased HGH levels. A number of the ingredients talked about in this book have shown tremendous benefit for people recovering from surgery or trauma.

Who should not take an HGH secretogogue?

It is my advice that anyone with active cancer or who has been in remission for at least 2 years should not try to increase their HGH levels. I also do not recommend an HGH secretogogue for people below the age of 25 unless they fall into one of the above categories (obesity, hysterectomy, chronic degenerative disease, etc.). In these cases a short course should be taken and evaluated for efficacy. HGH secretagogues are also not recommended during pregnancy or for nursing mothers.

Are there any other synergistic nutrients that can further enhance HGH levels?

Yes, I have written a book on three very powerful nutrients (Muramyl peptides, Beta 1,3-d-glucan, and calcium d-glucarate) that modulate the immune system and increase hormonal detoxification. I believe that these nutrients have a beneficial effect on HGH levels by clearing out the interfering foreign hormones from the body and allowing for a clearer "hormonal communication" to take place between the target tissue and the hypothalamus/pituitary complex. Please see www.AgeWellWithHGH.com for more information on these powerful nutrients.

What is the cost of taking an HGH Secretagogue?

Each product has its own cost, but the average cost of a good HGH secretogogue is anywhere from $65 to $80/ month. Before you tell me how expensive that is let's look at the daily cost and the benefits such a formula can make in your life. At $80/month an HGH secretogogue will cost you $2.58/day. Many people spend more than that on their morning latté at Starbucks and that coffee will not make you feel as good in the long run as a course of HGH raising secretogogue. When looking at whether or not you can afford to take a product like this you must evaluate the value you will be getting out of it. For many people the incredible sleep they get more than makes up for the cost. Put weight loss, increased mental clarity, energy and stamina, and increased sexual energy, and you can see the $80/month is well spent.

If I am taking a good HGH secretogogue, do I need to do anything about exercise, or my diet and lifestyle?

Taking an HGH raising secretogogue is only one way to naturally increase the output of HGH from your pituitary. In fact, you may only be getting some of the benefits of the HGH secretogogue if you don't make some simple changes in your diet and lifestyle, and begin to add in some exercise. Naturally raising HGH levels has a lot to do with finding a natural balance between factors that stimulate HGH production and factors that inhibit or prevent HGH release.

An HGH secretogogue naturally raises your HGH levels by providing stimulus to the hypothalamus to increase the output of GHRH, increasing the stimulation of GHRH to the pituitary, and providing the precursors for HGH production. It does this whilst leaving the regulatory processes in place. In most cases the regulatory processes are stronger than the influence of the HGH secretogogue. What do I mean by this? Well, let's say you are taking one of the newer targeted liposomal delivery HGH secretagogues, but do nothing to change your diet and lifestyle. You continue to eat a diet high in refined carbohydrates, drink coffee, and lead a stressful lifestyle. The HGH secretogogue you are taking is providing the stimulus to increase your HGH levels, but the diet and lifestyle are providing a much stronger inhibitory stimulus by increasing levels of the inhibitory hormone somatostatin that you are probably only getting a fraction of the benefits from the HGH secretogogue. If you want to get the most "bang for your buck" from your HGH secretogogue you would be well advised to implement some of the following exercise, diet, and lifestyle advice.

Benefits You May Experience Naturally Raising Your HGH Levels

1. Relief from chronic arthritis

2. Insomnia replaced with deep and restful sleep

3. Pain relief from auto-immune diseases such as lupus and rheumatoid arthritis

4. Resolution of chronic fatigue syndrome and Epstein Barr virus

5. Increased energy levels

6. Improved stamina throughout the day and during exercise

7. Increased recovery time when working out and lifting weights

8. Better skin

9. Resolution of old injuries

10. Increased mental clarity, improved memory, and resolution of dpression

11. Weight loss: Increased muscle mass and a loss of body fat

12. Hormonal regulation- more regular periods, fewer menopausal symptoms

13. Improved digestive function

CHAPTER SIX

ADDITIONAL WAYS TO ENHANCE HGH LEVELS IN THE BODY—EXERCISE, DIET, AND LIFESTYLE

The effectiveness of the third generation of HGH secretagogues lies with the advanced targeted liposomal delivery system and the presence of key nutrients that stimulate the pituitary to release its own stores of HGH and act as precursors for the synthesis of HGH. However, there are other factors at play that have a profound effect on the output of HGH from the pituitary. These include the following:

1. Regular exercise

2. A lifestyle that supports your anti-aging efforts

3. A diet that supports HGH function

The next section will deal with these three very important aspects of naturally raising your HGH levels as you age: Exercise, diet and lifestyle.

Exercise as a Way to Stimulate HGH Release

It is well known that exercise is a very strong trigger to increase HGH secretion. What is not so well know is that the higher the intensity of exercise the greater the effect on growth hormone output. One of the best ways to achieve a high intensity of exercise, and thus increase HGH levels, is to use the concept of interval training. Interval training combines short periods (15 – 90 seconds) of high intensity aerobic and anaerobic exercise at or near maximal intensity with periods of shorter lower-intensity exercise (1 – 3) minutes. At high rates of intensity the body produces greater and greater amounts of a substance called lactic acid. This begins to accumulate in the muscle and blood stream. The purpose of high intensity interval training is to push your body into what is called the "lactic acid threshold", which is the point at which the production of lactic acid exceeds the body's ability to clear it. Exercising above the lactic acid threshold is one of the strongest stimuli for growth hormone output from the pituitary. Research has shown that people who used interval training lost 9 times more fat than a similar group doing standard aerobic exercise, even though they exercised less than half of the time and expended 50% fewer calories during their exercise routine.

It is beyond the scope of this book to go into an in-depth study of interval training. We recommend that you visit our website www.AgeWellWithHGH.com for more information. However, I will detail some things you can do to make a tremendous difference in your HGH output.

Interval training is designed to burn fat, increase HGH output, build muscle, and lose weight. It combines high intensity aerobic exercise with high intensity anaerobic exercise into a seamless 30 minute full body work out. The effects of this type of workout are amazing. Growth hormone output will increase, and the fat burning effect can last up to two days post-workout.

A few caveats before starting any exercise program

1. A consultation with a physician is always recommended prior to beginning a new exercise program. If you are interested in such a program, you might want to show this section of the book to your health care provider.

2. Remember, it is important that you exercise at whatever level you choose, one that is appropriate for you.

3. Assess your current physical status and set realistic goals based on that.

4. In many experts' opinion over-training is worse than no training!

Timing of Exercise

It is important that you time your exercise program to coincide with the best time for HGH release in your body.

For instance, the lower your blood glucose levels are during exercise the greater the HGH spike you'll get post exercise. The low blood glucose forces your body to release HGH to stimulate the burning of fat for energy. The best time for HGH stimulating exercise is first thing in the morning after an all-night fast, and 30 minutes to one hour after taking any type of HGH stimulating secretagogues. If you cannot exercise first thing in the morning, time your exercise to take place 2-3 hours after your meal, so you can burn off the glucose from the meal before you workout. For the maximum HGH stimulation, fat burning, and weight loss you should do a fair amount of the aerobic exercise first. This will reduce your blood glucose levels and stimulate the secretion of HGH to begin the burning of fat for energy. Planning your workout in advance to take advantage of these factors will result in up to a 250% increase in HGH secretion. Eat a high protein, low carbohydrate and moderate fat meal 15 to 45 minutes after exercise in order to sustain the increase in HGH secretion. Remember the majority of the HGH will be turned into IGF-1, which will continue the beneficial effects of HGH for up to 20 hours after its formation in the liver.

HGH Releasing Exercises

The ideal HGH releasing exercise involves both anaerobic and aerobic exercise at a fairly high level of intensity for about 30 minutes 3 times/week. Over the course of 30 minutes you may have 5 short bouts of aerobic exercise mixed in with 5-6 short bouts of anaerobic exercise in the form of resistance training. These bouts flow together in a continuous program that is designed to have you exercising at a high intensity throughout the 30 minutes. For the sake of simplicity I will break the program down into its aerobic and anaerobic portions, and give you some examples of what you can do in each session. The exercise portion of my website, www.AgeWellWithHGH.com, has more information.

Aerobic portion

The aerobic portion of the program makes use of the stationery bicycle, the stair master, the treadmill, or the elliptical trainer. It uses the principle of exercise intervals to get the most benefit. The aerobic portions are punctuated by short amounts of higher, usually unsustainable amounts of exertion. This usually lasts for no more than one minute and puts the body into an anaerobic state, which increases the lactic acid threshold in the body, which is a very strong stimulus for HGH release. During the high intensity intervals you want to be exercising at a high intensity i.e. you are very short of breath and are pushing yourself very hard. Once the interval is complete you return to your former intensity for a few minutes before hitting another interval or move quickly into a short bout of anaerobic exercise.

Aerobic exercise is geared towards the movement of cellular fuel in the body, where it can be burned for energy and moved away from fuel storage. There is a shift in the hormonal output during aerobic exercise that allows this to take place. We see a decrease in hormones such as insulin, which are the primary storage hormones, and an increase in hormones such as growth hormone, which are the primary fuel mobilizing hormones.

It is important to use as many muscles as possible when doing the aerobics portion of the program. Too many aerobic exercises focus on the legs and leave out the upper body muscles. Using small free weights when on the treadmill or stationary bicycle can incorporate an upper body workout into your routine. Select a weight that will stretch you but not one that is too heavy that you cannot finish the exercise.

It is easy to design short aerobic exercises that incorporate intervals of high intensity workout. It is best to keep your aerobic bouts to under 4 minutes and to include at least 30 seconds of high intensity intervals for every 2 minutes of lesser aerobic exercise.

Please visit www.AgeWellWithHGH.com for a sample of aerobic exercise routines punctuated with short intervals of high intensity.

In summary, the aerobic portion of your exercise routine is designed to get you to exercise above the lactic acid threshold for short periods of time. This provides the stimuli to increase HGH levels and burn fat.

Anaerobic portion

The anaerobic portion of the program focuses on weight training, and incorporates the use of free weights, floor exercises, and resistance exercise machines. The primary hormone affected by weight training is growth hormone. Weight training's effect on growth hormone levels is dependent on factors such as the weight used, the number of repetitions, the number of sets, and the rest period in between the sets.

The basic principle of an anti-aging weight-training program uses light weights that are lifted slowly and completely to failure over the course of 10 to 12 reps. I recommend that you lift the weight over 4 – 5 seconds and return it to neutral in 1 second. Keep the weight moving at a consistent pace and return smoothly, i.e. don't just let it drop. Research has shown that controlled lifting speeds throughout the set will increase strength and muscle gain. The use of light weights with high repetition will decrease the likelihood of injury, and increase the lactic acid threshold in the muscles, which has been shown to be a strong stimulus for growth hormone release.

I also recommend that you incorporate free weights into your anaerobic routine. Use free weights as you do lunges across the room, and as you do star bursts or squats. The use of free weights will often increase your heart rate faster than aerobic exercise, so if you find that you are having a hard time getting your heart rate up, break off the aerobics machine and try some lunges across the room while doing biceps curls with free weights. You will find that this will increase your heart rate very nicely.

Again, it is beyond the scope of this book to go into a more in-depth discussion of weight training. Some people have never used weight machines or free weights before. For these people I recommend that you work with a certified professional before embarking on a weight training program to get some training in the use of this equipment so you can use it safely and effectively and reduce the likelihood of injuring yourself. For a sample routine of anaerobic exercise please visit the articles section at www.AgeWellWithHGH.com

Frequently Asked Questions about Exercising to Increase HGH Output

What benefits will I get from following this type of exercise routine?

By following a routine of 30 minutes of exercise that incorporates aerobic exercise and strength building anaerobic exercise you will experience a true cardiovascular work out, with improved muscle tone, increased lean muscle mass, increased body fat burning, general metabolic enhancement, and fat loss in one complete program. The aerobic portion is essential for fat loss and cardiovascular fitness, and the anaerobic exercise is essential for building lean muscle mass and increasing overall strength. The purpose of the high intensity is to push your body into what is called "the lactic acid threshold", which will increase the output of HGH by as much as 250%.

How often should I exercise per week?

I recommend that you do an exercise routine three times/ week. Half an hour three times/week is all you need to feel the amazing benefits of this type of exercise routine. However, you may wish to do the aerobic interval training portion a couple of times more during the week. Doing more than this will lead to overtraining, which can slow fat burning and muscle building.

Should I work with a trainer?

I recommend that you work with either a trainer or a partner who can be with you to help you keep you in a state of high intensity. Human nature prevents most of us from exercising at the highest rate if you are by yourself. I work out with my wife. She works with me for half an hour and then I work with her. It works very well.

What if I do not belong to a gym, can I still do this form of training?

This form of training is not limited to those with a gym membership. Any form of exercise can use the same principles of high intensity interval training. If you are a runner, commit to doing short sprints for a minute every 3-4 minutes during your run, or purchase some light free weights to take with you, or run where there are hills and do some fast hill running. This principle can be applied to cycling, swimming, fast walking, rowing.

One of the things that you may not be able to take advantage of is the anaerobic resistance portion of the training, which is an important part of the program. This is where the free weights can come in handy. You can often get free weights at local thrift stores. However, even without weights you can still do lunges, star squats, and other full-body exercise.

I don't want to ride a bike or run. Are there other forms of exercise that are considered interval training?

Yes, activities such as basketball, squash, racketball, or soccer should be classified as interval training because they are stop and start sports and incorporate short bouts of high intensity exercise.

What about taking time off?

Taking time off from training is known as detraining, and yes, you should regularly detrain. I recommend taking a week off for every 8 to 9 weeks of working out. This will give your body an excellent chance to recuperate and take advantage of all the tissue repair and muscle growth that takes place when growth hormone levels are elevated! It is interesting that growth hormone and testosterone output increase during detraining, which may explain why many people who come back to training after a week's absence have an increase in size and strength.

Additional Information

I have prepared a number of exercise related articles on my website www.AgeWellWithHGH.com. Please feel free to use them.

A lifestyle that supports your anti-aging efforts

The HGH raising abilities of HGH secretagogues are so effective that many people choose not to change their lifestyle because they feel so good. I am a great believer in motivating people to make the greatest change in their lives, which is why I am going to outline some lifestyle factors that can significantly improve not only your HGH levels but also your quality of life.

When you are spending money on a product to raise your HGH levels wouldn't you want to make the most of that investment by doing all you can to enhance its activity and minimize the things that would decrease its effectiveness? In the course of this book I have mentioned a few of the factors that cause your hypothalamus to preferentially increase the output of somatostatin (the HGH inhibitor) at the expense of GHRH (the HGH enhancer).

If you are serious about increasing HGH, remove all sources of toxicity in your body by quitting smoking, work to reduce and eliminate all drugs, prescription and otherwise, and limit the consumption of alcohol. By doing these you will more effectively raise your HGH levels, giving you the benefits of increased muscle mass, decreased body fat, improved tissue repair, and increased energy.

Stress is another factor that can have a strong impact on HGH release. Stress is the individual's generalized response to the varied demands of life. A certain degree of stress is helpful and enhances survival, while too much stress can be harmful and impair survival. Humans experience stress mentally, emotionally and physically from internal and external causes. Our bodies react to stress in much the same general way regardless of what's causing the stress. Intense or prolonged stress produces changes in the nervous system which causes the endocrine glands to release hormones that affect different tissues throughout the body. One of these hormones is called cortisol. Cortisol is a very strong inhibitor of HGH release. There are a number of wonderful ways to reduce stress that will benefit the output of HGH. I encourage you to read my article called "We're Hoping You're Coping" in the articles section of my website: www.AgeWellWithHGH.com

Having a high blood sugar level, another lifestyle factor that causes a decrease in HGH, will be covered in more depth in the diet section.

Sleep is extremely important for healthy secretion of HGH. In fact it has been said that sleep is an anti-aging activity! Your body repairs and rebuilds itself during sleep, which is why HGH secretion is at its highest level at night. You are increasing your aging when you don't get enough sleep.

There are a number of myths about sleep. One of these is that you need less sleep as you age. This is simply not true. You need just as much sleep when you are older as you did when you were younger. One of the problems is you lose the ability sleep well as you age. This may be due to decreasing levels of HGH. Many people who take one of the 3rd generation HGH secretagogue notice a profound improvement in their sleep.

Another myth is that you are getting enough sleep if you are not tired when you wake. This is not true because you may be running with higher levels of the stress hormone cortisol in the morning than normal.

I cannot stress more the importance of getting enough sleep. Sleep deprivation is one of the most important risk factors for accelerated aging. For more information, please see my article on sleep in the articles section of my website: www.AgeWellWithHGH.com.

Work on the Following Lifestyle Factors that Negatively Impact HGH Levels

1. Work to reduce toxicity in your body.

2. Reduce stress in your life.

3. Reduce high blood sugar levels.

4. Improve your sleep.

5. Have an exercise program that allows for appropriate recovery time and does not over exercise.

A Diet That Supports HGH Function

You might be surprised to hear me say that a healthy diet is the most effective way to prevent the effects of premature aging on the body. Of all the factors that influence our health, we have the greatest control over what we put in our body in the form of food and liquid. Yet most people make choices that speed the aging process.

1. Reduce or eliminate all forms of simple and refined sugars that cause HGH suppressing blood sugar swings

Problems with high blood sugar levels have reached an epidemic proportion in this country causing increasing levels of obesity and type II Diabetes in every age group from young kids to the elderly. In short, we need to avoid all sources of simple and refined sugars in our diets. If you were to do just this one thing, you would see rapid improvements in your health and well-being, and, over time, you would begin to lose weight, experience greater energy, mental focus, and stamina. It is interesting that the many benefits of removing simple and refined sugars from the diet mirror the benefits of higher HGH levels. This may have a lot to do with the HGH suppressing effects of blood sugar swings. I am not an advocate of the extremely low carbohydrate diets. Carbohydrate is a fuel, and as such we need moderate amounts of real carbohydrates to run our bodies.

These so-called real carbohydrates are found mostly in high fiber vegetables that grow above ground. They are the preferred carbohydrate of the body because they slow the release of simple carbohydrates such as glucose into the blood stream, and thus do not cause an increase in insulin level. Insulin is the hormone that pushes sugar into the cells thus lowering blood sugar levels. Unfortunately insulin is a very effective fat-forming hormone. It can easily turn carbohydrates into fat. High insulin levels, seen in diets that are constantly high in refined carbohydrates and sugars, cause you to gain weight, and also cause a decrease in HGH output from the pituitary. Some of the least beneficial carbohydrates to reduce or avoid include the following:

   a. Refined grains- white flour, bread, baked goods

   b. Sugars in all forms- table sugar, jams and jellies

   c. Starchy foods such as corn and potatoes

It is beyond the scope of this book to go into all of the reasons sugars and simple carbohydrates should be avoided. Please see the article on the effects of excess sugar consumption on human physiology in the articles section of my website: www.AgeWellWithHGH.com

2. Whole foods and minimal amounts of processed foods: plenty of nutrient dense foods consumed in balanced meals

You are what you digest and assimilate. Therefore, it is important to choose foods that can rebuild your proteins, fats, and carbohydrates on a continuous basis. These foods are best in their whole and unprocessed forms, i.e. foods that you can pick, gather, harvest, milk, hunt, or fish. Therefore, stay away from processed foods because they are likely to be damaged and full of toxins. Your diet should be composed of proteins, healthy fats, non-starchy vegetables and real carbohydrates. These are foods that are rich in the nutrients that can increase cellular and tissue repair, balance hormonal secretions, optimize brain function, and enhance proper tissue and muscle growth.

It is also important to make sure that you consume these in a ratio that allows for the most beneficial release of hormones. Eating a well balanced meal will keep your hormones balanced. For instance, you will increase your insulin levels if you eat too many carbohydrates, and you will increase your cortisol levels if you eat a diet too high in protein. Both of these have a detrimental effect on your HGH output. You should focus on eating at least three main meals/day. Try not to skip meals, which can cause problems with your HGH output.

A balanced meal is composed of the four main food groups: proteins, healthy fats, non-starchy vegetables, and real carbohydrates. To create a balanced meal, divide your plate into three sections and place proteins, real carbohydrates and non-starchy vegetables into each of these sections. The healthy fat can be added to all or some of the sections. For more details on the four elements of a balanced meal please

see the article section of my website:
www.AgeWellWithHGH.com

Summary of the Anti-Aging Diet

The diet that is relatively high in protein and low in carbohydrate will have the greatest benefit for HGH secretion. As the levels of carbohydrate decrease in the diet, hormones such as growth hormone start to increase and cortisol levels begin to decrease. Getting a balanced meal right every time is difficult, which is why I use and recommend the protein/carbohydrate ratio checklist (see the article on my website: www.AgeWellWithHGH.com for more details). Getting the correct protein to carbohydrate ratio will maximize the output of growth hormone from the pituitary.

Diet with the Most Beneficial Effect on Hormone Output

1. Reduce or eliminate all forms of sugar

2. Eat whole foods and minimal amounts of processed foods

3. Eat healthy sources of good protein

4. Consume plenty of sources of healthy fat

5. Choose real carbohydrates

6. Focus on non-starchy vegetables

For more information on an anti-aging diet please refer to these resources:

Books

Nourishing Traditions by Sally Fallon

Dr. Mercola's Total Health Cookbook & Program- Joseph Mercola, DO

The Schwarzbein Principle- Diana Schwarzbein, MD

The Schwarzbein Principle II- Diana Schwarzbein, MD

Websites

http://www.AgeWellWithHGH.com

http://www.Mercola.com

http://www.WestonPriceFoundation.com

SUMMARY

The information in this book may seem too good to be true, but the benefits you will experience when you naturally raise your growth hormone levels are real. It is possible to get these benefits by naturally raising their HGH levels either through the use of products that naturally increase HGH output, or by following an HGH friendly exercise, diet and lifestyle routine. When you finally deal with the reason your HGH levels drop as you age and begin to implement some of the changes to diet and lifestyle, coupled with the use of an HGH secretagogue, you can experience a return to the level of health, energy and vitality you had in your youth.

REFERENCES

Books

Guyton AC, Textbook of Medical Physiology- 8th edition. *W B Saunders Company*, Philadelphia 1991

Schwarzbein D, The Schwarzbein Principle II- The Transition. *Health Communications Inc,* Deerfield Beach 2002

Mercola J, et al. Dr. Mercola's Total Health Cookbook and Program, *Mercola.com*, Schaumberg 2004

Rubin JS, The Maker's Diet. *Siloam*, Lake Mary 2004

Murray M and Pizzorno J, Textbook of Natural Medicine-Revised 2nd edition. *Prima*, Rocklin 1998

Abstracts and research articles

Akhtar MK, et al. Antidiabetic evaluation of Mucuna pruriens, Linn seeds. *J Pak Med Assoc*. 1990 Jul;40(7):147-50.

Aleppo G, et al. Chronic L-alpha-glyceryl-phosphoryl-choline increases inositol phosphate formation in brain slices and neuronal cultures. *Pharmacol Toxicol*. 1994 Feb;74(2):95-100.

Altamyshev A. et al., What we know about Mumie" Moscow, 1989

Alving CR. Liposomes as carriers of antigens and adjuvants. *Immunol Methods*. 1991 Jun 24;140(1):1-13.

Amemta F. Del Valle M, Vega JA, Zaccheo D. Age-related structural changes in the rat cerebella cotrtex: effect of choline alfoscarate treatment. *Mech Aging Dev.* 1991; 61: 173-186

Amemta F. Del Valle M, Vega JA, Zaccheo D. long-term choline alfoscarate treatment counters age-dependent microanatomical changes in rat brains. *Prog Neuropsychopharmacol boil Psychiatyr. I1994; 18:915-924*

Bando H, et al Impaired secretion of growth hormone-releasing hormone, growth hormone and IGF-I in elderly men. *Acta Endocrinol (Copenh)*. 1991 Jan;124(1):31-6

Bazzare, T, Nutrition and strength in nutrition in exercise and sport *CRC press*, Boca Raton, 1998

Bhattacharya SK, et al.Adaptogenic activity of Siotone, a polyherbal formulation of Ayurvedic rasayanas. *Indian J Exp Biol*. 2000 Feb;38(2):119-28.

Bhaumik, S et al. *Phytotherapy Res.*, 1993; vol. 7

Blomqvist BI., et al Glutamine and alpha-ketoglutarate prevent the decrease in muscle free glutamine concentration and influence protein synthesis after total hip replacement. *Metabolism: Clinical & Experimental*. 44(9):1215-22, 1995 Sep.

Blomstrand, E., et al., Effect of Branch Chained Amino Acid supplementation on the exercise-induced change in aromatic amino acid concentration in human muscle. *Acta physiol Scand..* 146:293-298

Boucher, L. et al., Ornithine alpha ketoglutarate modulates protein metabolism in burn injured rats. *American Jo Physiology*. 1997, 273 (3):557-63

Boyd A., et al. Stimulation of growth hormone secretion by L-dopa *New England Jounal of Medicine,* 1970, 283:1425

Brabagello Sanglorgi G et al., Alpha-Glycerylphosphorylcholine in the mental recovery of cerebral ischemic attacks. An Italian multicenter clinical trial. *Ann NY Acad Sci* 1994 June 30;717:253-69

Bricon, T. et al., Ornithine alpha ketoglutarate metabolism after eneral administration in burn patients. *American Jo Clin Nut*. 1997, 65(2):512-18

Bucci LR. Selected herbals and human exercise performance. *Am J Clin Nutr*. 2000 Aug;72(2 Suppl):624S-36S

Bucci, Luke, Ph.D., Nutrients as Ergogenic Aids for Sports and Exercise. *CRC Press*, Boca Raton 1993, pgs. 69 & 72

Canal N., Effect of L-alpha-glyceryl-phosphorylcholine on amnesia caused by scopolamine. *Int J Clin Pharmacol Ther Toxicol*. 1991 Mar;29(3):103-7.

Ceda GP, Ceresini G. Denti., et al, Alpha Glycerylphosphorylcholine administration increases the GH response to GHRH of young and elderly subjects. *Horm metab Res.* 1992;24: 119-121

Christina Schneid, et al. In vivo induction of insulin secretion by ornithine [alpha]-ketoglutarate: Involvement of nitric oxide and glutamine. *Metabolism*, 52 (3): 344-350, 2003 Mar.

Clin invest, 97 (5):1319-28, 1996, March

Cordido F, et al, Cholinergic receptor activation by pyridostigmine restores growth hormone (GH) responsiveness to GH-releasing hormone administration in obese subjects: evidence for hypothalamic somatostatinergic participation in the blunted GH release of obesity. *J Clin Endocrinol Metab*. 1989 Feb;68(2):290-3.

Cynober LA Ornithine Alpha-Ketoglutarate in nutritional support. *Nutrition* 7(5):313-321, 1991 sept/Oct

Cynober LA, The use of alpha-ketoglutarate salts in clinical nutrition and metabolic care. *Current Opinion in Clinical Nutrition & Metabolic Care*. 2(1):33-7, 1999 Jan.

Devesa J, et al Regulation of hypothalamic somatostatin by glucocorticoids. *J Steroid Biochem Mol Biol*. 1995 Jun;53(1-6):277-82.

Donati L, et al. Nutritional and clinical efficacy of ornithine alpha-ketoglutarate in severe burn patients. *Clin Nutr*. 1999 Oct;18(5):307-11.

Drago F, et al. Behavioral effects of l-alpha-glycerylphosphorylcholine :influence on cognitive mechanisms in the rat. *Pharmacol biochem behave* 1992 Feb;41(2):445-8

Duranton B, et al. Preventive administration of ornithine alpha-ketoglutarate improves intestinal mucosal repair after transient ischemia in rats. *Crit Care Med.* 1998 Jan;26(1):120-5.

Ghigo E, et al. Arginine potentiates but does not restore the blunted growth hormone response to growth hormone-releasing hormone in obesity. *Metabolism.* 1992 May;41(5):560-3.

Ghigo E, et al., Growth hormone (GH) responsiveness to combined administration of arginine and GH-releasing hormone does not vary with age in man. *J Clin Endocrinol Metab.* 1990 Dec;71(6):1481-5

Ghosal S., et. Al, *Phytotherapy Res.* 1991, 5,211

Gillberg P. et al, Two years of treatment with recombinant growth hormone increases bone mineral density in men with idiopathic osteoporosis. *J Clin Endocrinol Metab* 200;87:4900-4906

Giusti, M et al. Effect of cholinergic tone on growth hormone-releasing hormone-induced secretion of growth hormone in normal aging. *Aging (Milano).* 1992 Sep;4(3):231-7

Giustina A, et al. Arginine normalizes the growth hormone (GH) response to GH-releasing hormone in adult patients receiving chronic daily immunosuppressive glucocorticoid therapy. *J Clin Endocrinol Metab.* 1992 Jun;74(6):1301-5.

Goel RK, et al Antiulcerogenic and antiinflammatory studies with shilajit. *J Ethnopharmacol.* 1990 Apr;29(1):95-103

Goldberg,I.(1980).L-Tyrosine in Depression. *Lancet* , 2 , 364.

Grover JK, et al. Traditional Indian anti-diabetic plants attenuate progression of renal damage in streptozotocin induced diabetic mice. *Int J Food Sci Nutri.* 201 Jan;52(1)79-82

Grover, JK, et al. Medicinal plants of India with anti-diabetic properties *J Ethnopharmacol.* 2002 Jun;81(1):81-100.

Hanew K, et al The inhibitory effects of growth hormone-releasing hormone (GHRH)-antagonist on GHRH, L-dopa, and clonidine-induced GH secretion in normal subjects. *J Clin Endocrinol Metab.* 1996 May;81(5):1952-5.

Hares, P et al., Effect of ornithine alpha ketoglutarate (OAKG) on the response of brain metabolism to hypoxia in the dog. *Stroke* 1978 May-Jun;9(3):222-4

Indian Journal of Pharmacology 1992, vol 24

J Am Coll Cardiol 2002;39:37-48

Jeevanandam M. Holaday NJ. Petersen SR., Ornithine-alpha-ketoglutarate (OKG) supplementation is more effective than its component salts in traumatized rats. *Journal of Nutrition.* 126(9):2141-50, 1996 Sep.

Journal of Ethnopharmacology, 1990, vol. 29

Kelly, Gregory, Textbook of natural Medicine, edited by Pizzorno, J., Murray, M., *Churchill Livingston,* 1999, Chapter 59, 521-541

Koppeschaar HP, et al. Differential effects of arginine on growth hormone releasing hormone and insulin induced growth hormone secretion. *Clin Endocrinol (Oxf).* 1992 May;36(5):487-90

Koppeschaar, et al., *Clinical Endocrinology,* Volume 36, #5 1992 May

Laborit, H, Sodium 4-hydroxybutyrate. *Inter Jo Neuropharmacology, 1964, 3:433-52*

Lang I, et al Effects of sex and age on growth hormone response to growth hormone-releasing hormone in healthy individuals. *J Clin Endocrinol Metab.* 1987 Sep;65(3):535-40.

Le Boucher J, et al. Modulation of immune response with ornithine A-ketoglutarate in burn injury: an arginine or glutamine dependency? *Nutrition.* 1999 Oct;15(10):773-7

Le Boucher, J et al. Ornithine alpha Ketoglutarate: the puzzle. *Nutrition* 14:870-873, 1998

Leal-Cerro A, et al Effect of enhancement of endogenous cholinergic tone with pyridostigmine on growth hormone (GH) responses to GH-releasing hormone in patients with Cushing's syndrome. *Clin Endocrinol (Oxf)*. 1990 Aug;33(2):291-5.

Lieberman MD, et al.; Enhancement of interleukin-2 immunotherapy with l-arginine. *Annals of Surgery,* 1992 Feb, 215(2):157-65

Lopez CM, et al. Effect of a new cognition enhancer, alpha-glycerylphosphorylcholine, on scopolamine-induced amnesia and brain acetylcholine. *Pharmacol biochem behave* 1991 Aug;39(4):835-40

Ma Q., et al. Effect of supplemental L-arginine in a chemical-induced model of colorectal cancer *World J Surg* 1996 Oct;20(8):1087-91

Manayam BV, et al. Effect of antiparkinson drug HP-200 (Mucuna pruriens) on the central monoaminergic neurotransmitters. *Phytother Res.* 2004 Feb;18(2):97-101

Mazza E, et al. Effect of the potentiation of cholinergic activity on the variability in individual GH response to GH-releasing hormone. *J Endocrinol Invest.* 1989 Dec;12(11):795-8

Meyers,S.(2000).Use of Neurotransmitter Precursors for Treatment of Depression. *Altern Med Rev* , 5 (1) , 64-71.

Mitsuhashi S, et al. Effect of oral administration of L-dopa on the plasma levels of growth hormone-releasing hormone

(GHRH) in normal subjects and patients with various endocrine and metabolic diseases. *Nippon Naibunpi Gakkai Zasshi.* 1987 Aug 20;63(8):934-46

Moinard, C., et al. Involvement of glutamine, arginine, and polyamines in the action of ornithine alpha-ketoglutarate on macrophage functions in stressed rats. *J Leukoc Biol.* 2000 Jun;67(6):834-40

Muller EE, et al. Somatotropic dysregulation in old mammals. *Horm Res.* 1995;43(1-3):39-45

Nagashayana N et al., Association of L-dopa with recovery following ayurvedic medication for Parkinson's disease. *Adv Neurol* 199;80:565-74

Neri,D.;Wiegmann,D.;Stanny,R. et al. (1995).The effects of tyrosine on cognitive performance during extended wakefulness. *Avit Space Environ Med.* , 66 , 313–319.

Page MD, et al Growth hormone (GH) responses to arginine and L-dopa alone and after GHRH pretreatment. *Clin Endocrinol (Oxf).* 1988 May;28(5):551-8.

Parnetti L et al., Multicenter study of l-alpha-glycerylphosphorylcholine vs ST2000 among patients with senile dementia of alzhemier's type. *Drugs Aging.* 1993; Mar – April; 3, (2):159-64

Penalva A, et al. Activation of cholinergic neurotransmission by pyridostigmine reverses the inhibitory effect of hyperglycemia on growth hormone (GH) releasing hormone-induced GH secretion in man: does acute hyperglycemia act through hypothalamic release of somatostatin? *Neuroendocrinology.* 1989 May;49(5):551-4.

Penalva A, et al. Effect of enhancement of endogenous cholinergic tone with pyridostigmine on the dose-response relationships of growth hormone (GH)-releasing hormone-induced GH secretion in normal subjects. *J Clin Endocrinol Metab.* 1990 Feb;70(2):324-7.

Prakash D, et al. Some nutritional properties of the seeds of three Mucuna species. *Int J Food Sci Nutr.* 2001 Jan;52(1):79-82

Ricci A, Bronzenti E, Vega JA, Amenta F. Oral choline alfoscerate counteracts age-dependent loss of mossy fibers in the rat hippocampus. *Mech Aging Dev.* 1992; 66: 81-91

Roch-Arveiller M, et al. Ornithine alpha-ketoglutarate counteracts the decrease of liver cytochrome P-450 content in burned rats. *Nutrition.* 1999 May;15(5):379-83. Dumas, F. et al. Enteral ornithine alpha-ketoglutarate enhances intestinal adaptation to massive resection in rats. *Metabolism.* 1998 Nov;47(11):1366-71.

Sabelli,H.;Fawcett,J.;Gusovsky,F. et al.(1986).Clinical studies on the phenylethylamine hypothesis of affective disorder:urine and blood phenylacetic acid and phenylalanine dietary supplements. *Journal of Clinical Psychiatry* , 47 , 66–70.

Schena, F., Branched Chain Amino Acid supplementation during trekking at high altitude. *European Journal of Applied Physiology.* 65:394-398

Schliebs R, et al Systemic administration of defined extracts from Withania somnifera (Indian Ginseng) and Shilajit differentially affects cholinergic but not glutamatergic and GABAergic markers in rat brain. *Neurochem Int.* 1997 Feb;30(2):181-90

Schneid C, Darquy S, Cynober L, Reach G, De Bandt JP., Effects of ornithine alpha-ketoglutarate on insulin secretion in rat pancreatic islets: implication of nitric oxide synthase and glutamine synthetase pathways. *Br J Nutr. 2003* Feb;89(2):249-57.

Sharoerov I.S., Mumie and vitality of life Tashkent University, 1978

Singhal B, Lalkaka J, Sankhla C. Epidemiology and treatment of Parkinson's disease in India. *Parkinsonism Relat Disord.* 2003 Aug;9 Suppl 2:S105-9

Takahara, J et al., Stimulatory effects of gamma hydroxybutyric acid on growth hormone and prolactin release in humans. *Journal of Clinical Endocrinology and Metabolism.* 1977, 44:1014

Tiwari P, et al. Effects of Shijalit (Mumie) on the development of tolerance to morphine in mice *Phytother Res* 2001 15(2):177-179

Toricelli P, et al. L-arginine and L-lysine stimulation on cultured osteoblasts. *Biomed Parmacother* 2002;56:492-497

Tripathi YB, et al. Effect of the alcohol extract of the seeds of Mucuna pruriens on free radicals and oxidative stress in albino rats. *Phytother Res*. 2002 Sep;16(6):534-8.

Tripathi YB, et al. Effects of alcohol extract of the seeds of Mucuna pruriens on free radicals and oxidative stress in albino rats. *Jo Ethnopharm* 2002 June;81(1):81-100

Valcavi R, et al. Effects of oral glucose administration on spontaneous and growth hormone (GH)-releasing hormone-stimulated GH release in children and adults. *J Clin Endocrinol Metab*. 1994 Oct;79(4):1152-7.

Van Cauter, E et al., Simultaneous stimulation of slow wave sleep and growth hormone secretion by gamma hydroxybutyric acid in normal young men. *Journal of Clinical Investigation*. 1997, August 1 100(3):745-53

Welbourne T. Increased plasma bicarbonate and growth hormone after oral Glutamine load. *American Journal of Clinical Nutrition*. 1995; 61:1058-61

Wojcik,J. y Falk,W.(1990). Tyrosine for depression :a double-blind trial. *J Affect Disord*, 19, 125-132.

Yance D, Tabachnik B, Breakthrough Solutions: Adaptogenic botanical agents with anabolic/anti-catabolic actions for: stress resistance, lean muscle enhancement, cellular and systemic energy, and endocrine resuscitation. *Designs for health institute: #2*

Yance D, Tabachnik B, Breakthrough Solutions: The New Generation of Nutritional Agents for Stress Resistance, Energy, lean Muscle Enhancement, and Total Wellness. *Designs for health institute: #4*

Young,S.(1996).Behavioral effects of dietary neurotransmitter precursors : Basic and clinical aspects. *Neurosci Biobehav Rev*, 20 , 313-323. Wojcik,J. y Falk,W.(1990). Tyrosine for depression :a double-blind trial. *J Affect Disord*, 19, 125-132.

Yance D, Tabachnik B, Breakthrough Solutions: Adaptogenic botanical agents with anabolic/anti-catabolic actions for: stress resistance, lean muscle enhancement, cellular and systemic energy, and endocrine resuscitation. *Designs for health institute: #2*

Yance D, Tabachnik B, Breakthrough Solutions: The New Generation of Nutritional Agents for Stress Resistance, Energy, lean Muscle Enhancement, and Total Wellness. *Designs for health institute: #4*

Young,S.(1996).Behavioral effects of dietary neurotransmitter precursors : Basic and clinical aspects. *Neurosci Biobehav Rev*, 20 , 313-323.